OXFORD MEDICAL PUBLIC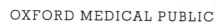

Immunizing Children

PRACTICAL GUIDES FOR GENERAL PRACTICE

1. *Cervical screening: a practical guide*
   Ann McPherson
2. *A basic formulary for general practice*
   G. B. Grant, D. A. Gregory, and T. D. van Zwanenberg
3. *Radiology*
   Robert F. Bury
4. *Stroke*
   Derick T. Wade
5. *Alcohol problems*
   P. D. Anderson, P. Wallace, and H. A. Jones
6. *Breast cancer screening*
   Joan Austoker and John Humphreys
7. *Computers: a guide to choosing and using*
   A. W. Willis and T. I. Stewart
8. *Immunizing children*
   Sue Sefi and J. A. Macfarlane

Forthcoming

Non-insulin-dependent diabetes
Ann-Louise Kinmonth
Screening tests used in child health surveillance
J. A. Macfarlane and Sue Sefi
Hypertension
T. Schofield

Immunizing Children

Practical Guides for General Practice   8

SUE SEFI
Health Visitor, Oxford

and

AIDAN MACFARLANE
Consultant Community Paediatrician, Oxford

Oxford   New York   Tokyo
OXFORD UNIVERSITY PRESS
1989

Oxford University Press, Walton Street, Oxford OX2 6DP

Oxford New York Toronto
Delhi Bombay Calcutta Madras Karachi
Petaling Jaya Singapore Hong Kong Tokyo
Nairobi Dar es Salaam Cape Town
Melbourne Auckland

and associated companies in
Berlin Ibadan

Oxford is a trade mark of Oxford University Press

Published in the United States
by Oxford University Press, New York

British Library Cataloguing in Publication Data
Sefi, Sue
Immunizing children.
1. Medicine. Immunisation
I. Title II. Macfarlane, Aidan
614.4'7
ISBN 0–19–261829–6

Library of Congress Cataloging in Publication Data
Sefi, Sue.
Immunizing children.
(Practical guides for general practice; 8)
(Oxford medical publications)
Bibliography. Includes index.
1. Immunization of children. I. Macfarlane, Aidan,
1939– . II. Title. III. Series. IV. Series:
Oxford medical publication. [DNLM: 1. Immunization—in
infancy & childhood. W1 PR141NK no. 8/WS 135 S453i]
RJ240.S44   1989   614.4'7'088054   88–31261
ISBN 0–19–261829–6

Typeset by Cotswold Typesetting Limited, Cheltenham
Printed in Great Britain
at the University Printing House, Oxford
by David Stanford
Printer to the University

Acknowledgements

We would like to thank the members of the 'Oxford Community Immunisation Group', listed below, for all their help and co-operation in the preparation of this manual.

Professor E. R. Moxon, Professor of Paediatrics, John Radcliffe Hospital

Dr J. A. Macfarlane, Consultant Community Paediatrician, Community Health Offices, Radcliffe Infirmary

Dr R. Mayon-White, Community Physician, Manor House, Headington

Dr G. Sleight, Senior Clinical Medical Officer, Community Health Offices, Radcliffe Infirmary

Dr D. Isaacs, Wellcome Trust Lecturer, Department of Paediatrics, John Radcliffe Hospital

Dr S. Dobson, University Clinical Lecturer in Paediatrics, John Radcliffe Hospital

Dr G. Tudor-Williams, Clinical Medical Officer, Department of Paediatrics, John Radcliffe Hospital

Mrs J. Moreton, Health Visitor, Kennington Health Centre, Oxford

Miss J. Frankland, Health Visitor, Department of Paediatrics, John Radcliffe Hospital

Mrs S. Sefi, Research and Resource Officer, Community Health Offices, Radcliffe Infirmary

We would also like to thank

Mrs V. A. Moar, Departmental Administrator, Department of Paediatrics, John Radcliffe Hospital

Thanks and acknowledgement are also due to the Department of Child Health, University of Nottingham, and the Child Health Section, Community Unit, Nottingham Health Authority, who, with Angus Nicol, have pioneered so much educational material.

Contents

Introduction   viii

1 Why we immunize   1

2 Immunization schedules   10

3 Absolute contra-indications for immunization   13

4 Special considerations for immunization   15

5 Immunization procedure   19
    History-taking   19
    Consent   20
    Giving the immunization   20
    Recording   23
    Storing vaccines   23
    Obtaining information   24

6 Reactions to immunization   25

7 Common problems   28

8 Comments parents may make   32

9 Future immunization targets   34

Appendices

A References and further reading   35

B Child resuscitation pack   37

C Check-list for home immunization   38

Index   39

Introduction

The immunization of children is the single most cost-effective form of prevention. Protecting children against infectious diseases is however achieved by two separate and essential steps. The first step is the development of safe and effective vaccines and the second is giving the vaccine to the entire population at risk.

To achieve this second step all professionals must be both knowledgeable about the procedures and confident about the benefits. Only then can they pass on accurate and reliable information to parents, allowing them to then make a properly informed decision.

This working manual has been specifically written so as to ensure the proper completion of this second step. It is in line with the DHSS guidelines, but is written in a practical and easily accessible form.

It is for those 'in the field' directly responsible for giving immunizations—general practitioners, health visitors, school nurses, practice nurses, clinical medical officers, and district nurses. It is also written so as to be understandable by parents.

To be adaptable for local use spaces have been left for you to fill in the following information:

your local immunization schedules on pages 10–11;
your local phone numbers showing who you should contact about queries on 'form' completion on page 23;
your local phone numbers showing who to contact with queries concerning an immunization problem on page 24.

Amongst much other essential information are sections giving the answers to the most common problems and to the questions most frequently asked by parents.

1 Why we immunize

We immunize children to prevent them suffering from serious infections. Active immunization can be defined as giving a modified antigen to provoke an antibody response so that the child develops immunity to that antigen.

Immunization is a positive health benefit to children. At a Royal College of Nursing conference on immunization against infectious disease in May 1986 it was stated that it is 'every child's right to be immunized'. The World Health Organization, in its document *Health for all* has clearly stated its aim of eradicating throughout Europe, by the year 2000, poliomyelitis, measles, neonatal tetanus, congenital rubella, and diphtheria.

Enthusiastic and knowledgeable health workers can achieve very high immunization levels in the communities in which they work (Begg and White 1987). Immunization uptake levels can be used as a measure of the effectiveness of the primary health care team, as each member delivers consistent advice, and contributes to the smooth running of a co-ordinated service.

Immunization offers protection to the individual, prevents substantial outbreaks of infectious disease, and in the case of smallpox, for instance, has led to the world-wide eradication of a serious, lethal disease. With high levels of immunization uptake, a 'herd immunity' is achieved, which helps protect those few children who cannot be immunized.

The present immunization policy in the UK, if followed, prevents a child from suffering from the following diseases:

- diphtheria,
- pertussis (whooping cough),
- tetanus (lockjaw),
- polio,

1

- measles,
- mumps (from autumn 1988),
- rubella (German measles),
- tuberculosis (selective immunization in some health authorities).

All children in the USA are required to have completed their immunization course before starting school. The UK policy, however, has maintained that immunization of children is a matter for parental choice. It is therefore the responsibility of all health workers to ensure that parents are given correct and up-to-date information, to enable them to choose wisely.

As information on immunization changes, and becomes more exact, health workers must keep up to date, and be prepared to change some of their own views and advice to parents. In the 1960s, for instance, one misconception was that asthma and eczema were contra-indications to giving pertussis immunization. It is important for health workers to recognize that contra-indications may change.

Every child eligible for immunization should be offered that protection. All the diseases that we immunize against may have severe consequences for those who are unprotected.

Diphtheria

In 1940, just before the introduction of diphtheria vaccine, there were 46 281 cases of diphtheria, with 2480 notified deaths. By 1957 the figures had dropped to 37 cases, with 6 notified deaths. During 1979–86 26 cases, with 1 death, were reported.

Although there has been a dramatic fall in incidence and mortality, immunization levels for diphtheria must be kept above 95 per cent. The causative organism may be present in some symptomless carriers, and cannot be eradicated.

Diphtheria is caused by a bacterium, *Corynebacterium diphtheriae*, which produces a toxin that inflames the membranes of the nose and throat, blocking the larynx and so obstructing the airways. Antibiotics are effective but if antitoxin is not given quickly a toxin produced by the bacterium will attack the heart and nervous system.

Complications include:

- heart damage,
- paralysis (which may recover),
- death (in up to 10 per cent of all cases, the 1–4 years age group being the most vulnerable).

Tetanus

Tetanus vaccine was introduced into the basic course of immunization of infants in 1961. From 1960 to 1969, 200–300 cases (all age groups), with about 27 associated deaths, a year, were reported in England and Wales. Notifications have since fallen to around 20 cases a year. Between 1981 and 1986 there were 62 notifications, only three of which involved children under 15 years of age.

Tetanus spores are present in soil, and enter the body after injury, often through a puncture wound, wounds contaminated by dirt or splinters, or wounds caused by burns. The wound may be trivial or unnoticed, such as a skin puncture caused by a rose thorn. Toxin from the anaerobic tetanus bacilli (*Clostridium tetani*) causes painful muscle spasms.

Complications include:

- lockjaw,
- painful muscular spasms,
- death (rare).

Pertussis (whooping cough)

In the early 1950s, the average annual number of cases of whooping cough reported was above 100 000, with a death rate of 1 in every 1000. In the 10 years after introduction of pertussis vaccine in 1957, this number fell to less than 30 000. In 1974 when immunization rates were over 80 per cent only 10 000 cases were reported. However, in the same year Kulenkampff *et al.* published the results of a study of 36 children admitted to hospital with severe neurological illness, 33 of whom had received pertussis vaccine during the week preceding onset of illness. The report referred to possible risk factors associated with the vaccine, although the study did not include a control group. Widespread publicity of this report, which appeared to question the safety of pertussis vaccine, resulted in a dramatic decline in immunized children. Only 3 out of every 10 children born in 1976 had been immunized against pertussis two years later. In consequence two major epidemics of whooping cough occurred, the first in 1977-9, with over 100 000 cases and 36 deaths in the UK, and the second in 1982, with almost 66 000 cases and 14 deaths in England and Wales (OHE 1984). Immunization rates since 1979 have begun to rise steadily as confidence in the benefits of vaccination has returned. More recent research, such as the National Childhood Encephalopathy Study (DHSS 1981), and also the Loveday judgment (Lancet 1988) have confirmed the efficacy and safety of the vaccine.

Whooping cough is caused by the highly communicable bacterium, *Bordetella pertussis*, which primarily affects the trachea and bronchi, resulting in episodes of paroxysmal coughing and vomiting, which can last for over six weeks. The child is infectious for three weeks unless an antibiotic such as erythromycin is given. This will not lessen the illness but is said to reduce the infectious period to five days (Harvey and Kovar 1985). A full course of vaccine (three doses) confers protection in over 80 per cent of recipients.

Complications include:

- convulsions,
- pneumonia,
- lung damage,
- temporary and/or permanent brain damage,
- subconjunctival haemorrhage,
- death (especially in babies aged less than six months).

Poliomyelitis

Routine vaccination began in 1956, using inactivated polio-myelitis vaccine (IPV; Salk). This was replaced in 1962 with oral, live attenuated vaccine (OPV; Sabin). Notifications of paralytic poliomyelitis have dropped from nearly 4000 in 1955 to 257 in 1960. Between 1974 and 1978 35 cases were reported. Notifications have averaged three per year since 1979.

Poliovirus, of which there are three types (I, II, and III), damages nerve cells. Man is its only natural host, carrying the virus in the intestine and spreading it by faecal con-tamination of hands, food, or water. An epidemic can quickly occur in an unprotected community.

Complications include:

- meningitis,
- temporary or permanent paralysis,
- death.

*Measles

Until the introduction of measles vaccine in 1968 the average annual number of cases varied between 160 000 and 800 000. In 1968 there were 90 deaths from measles. By the mid-1970s the annual number of cases had dropped to 50 000–180 000. Since 1970, an average of 13 children have died each year from measles or its complications.

Although the vaccine offers 95 per cent protection, and is safe, take up of the vaccine has been disappointingly low. National immunization figures for measles have never exceeded 65 per cent (Miller 1983; Begg and White 1987).

This is surprising, as measles is a highly contagious viral disease, which can cause complications in about 10 per cent of all cases. More rarely, serious neurological complications occur (about 1 in 2000 cases). This includes acute encephalitis, which can cause permanent brain damage, and more rarely, subacute sclerosing panencephalitis.

In contrast, since 1982, the USA has achieved an immunization level of 97 per cent of all children entering school. In 1983, 1436 notifications of measles were recorded for the USA as a whole, whereas in England and Wales notifications exceeded 97 000 (Wells 1987).

Complications include:

- otitis media,
- pneumonia,
- febrile convulsions,
- encephalitis,
- subacute sclerosing panencephalitis,
- death.

*Mumps

Until 1988 no vaccine against mumps was available in the UK. Mumps is caused by a paramyxovirus, and is transmitted by droplet spread from infected saliva. It causes swelling of one or both parotid glands.

Complications include:

- meningitis,
- encephalitis (about 1:400 cases),
- orchitis (30 per cent of adult cases),
- sensorineural hearing loss,
- pancreatitis (rare).

*Rubella (German measles)

The rubella virus was identified in 1962. Live attenuated rubella virus vaccine has been offered to schoolgirls aged 10–14 years, since 1970. It induces an antibody response in 95 per cent of those immunized and offers long-term protection.

If rubella is contracted during early pregnancy, especially during the first 10 weeks of gestation, it can result in fetal damage in up to 90 per cent of cases, causing severe abnormalities in the unborn baby (congenital rubella syndrome).

The baby may be stillborn, or suffer from one or more of the following handicaps:

- blindness,
- deafness (or impaired hearing),
- heart damage,
- mental retardation.

*From October 1988, a combined, single-dose vaccine against measles, mumps and rubella (MMR), was introduced in the UK with the aim of eliminating measles, mumps, and congenital rubella syndrome. To achieve this at least 90 per cent of all pre-school children should receive the vaccine. Girls aged 10–14 years will continue to receive rubella vaccine.

Tuberculosis

Routine vaccination of children with BCG vaccine against tuberculosis was introduced in the 1950s, although a marked decline in notifications and deaths from the disease was already occurring. The vaccine is over 70 per cent effective and gives protection for at least 15 years. The incidence of tuberculosis has continued to decline, from 117 000 notifications of cases and almost 50 000 deaths in 1913, to less than 1000 deaths in 1978 (Harvey and Kovar 1985). Although tuberculosis is now much less common it remains an important cause of morbidity and mortality, and the case fatality rate is above 10 per cent.

Tuberculosis (TB) is commonly caused by the organism *Mycobacterium tuberculosis*, and is acquired through airborne transmission from an infected person, often a member of the same household.

Later complications may include:

- infections of the lymph nodes,
- bronchiectasis and empyema,
- tuberculous meningitis,
- tuberculous peritonitis,
- tuberculous bones and joints,
- renal tuberculosis (rare).

Health districts have adopted different vaccination policies for tuberculosis. The majority, at present, continue to offer routine vaccination to all children aged 10–14 years, who have been shown to be tuberculin-negative following Mantoux or Heaf testing.

Other health districts, such as Oxfordshire, have discontinued routine vaccination of schoolchildren, and offer vaccination on a selective basis.

All health districts selectively vaccinate new-born babies of families with a history or high risk of TB. These babies should receive BCG (Bacille–Calmette–Guerin), intradermally, administered either in the maternity hospital, or, if born at home, by the health visitor. A Heaf test is not necessary. All household contacts of patients with sputum-positive pulmonary tuberculosis should also be tested and appropriate action taken.

A Heaf test uses the Heaf 'gun' to produce a circle of six small punctures, after tuberculin PPD (protein purified derivative) solution has been applied to a small area of skin surface, usually the inner forearm. The Heaf test is performed before vaccination, and is read 3–10 days later, by the school nurse, health visitor, or GP.

Reading a Heaf test

Result	Action
Negative	
Nothing to see, or, ≤3 raised papules	Not immune, vaccinate with BCG if a child
Positive	
Grade 1: 4+ raised papules	As above
Grade 2: raised red ring with joined papules	Refer for chest X-ray and medical opinion, unless BCG was previously given
Grade 3: raised red lump	Refer for chest X-ray and
Grade 4: vesiculated red lump	medical opinion

Note: individuals who are HIV-positive should *not* receive BCG vaccine.

2 Immunization schedules

Recommended national immunization schedule

Primary immunization

Birth   —BCG for some babies of migrant families, and those in contact with TB
3 months   —polio+diphtheria/tetanus/pertussis (triple)
$4\frac{1}{2}$-5 months —polio+diphtheria/tetanus/pertussis
$8\frac{1}{2}$-11 months —polio+diphtheria/tetanus/pertussis
12-18 months—measles/mumps/rubella (from 1.10.88)

Secondary immunization

4-5 years   —polio+diphtheria/tetanus

Tertiary immunization

10-14 years   —rubella (girls only)
10-14 years   —BCG (allow 3 weeks between BCG and rubella)
15-18 years   —polio+tetanus

All children should be immunized even if they present outside the recommended ages. No opportunity to immunize should be missed.

Local district immunization schedule

The local district immunization schedule for_____ is:

D/T/P and polio	1st dose	....
D/T/P and polio	2nd dose	....
D/T/P and polio	3rd dose	....

MMR   ....
D/T and polio   ....
Rubella   ....
BCG   ....
Tetanus and polio   ....

Other schedules

If the child has arrived from overseas and is staying in the UK, change to health district schedule. If there is doubt about which, if any, immunizations have been given, start a complete immunization programme. If the child is returning abroad within one year, keep to the foreign schedule.

Delays in the immunization programme

If immunizations have been delayed the gaps between giving the immunizations are:

- 6-8 weeks between the first two immunizations of polio+DTP. If whooping cough is prevalent, the interval between doses can be reduced to 4 weeks.
- Allow 4-6 months between 2nd and 3rd polio+DTP. If the primary course is interrupted it should be resumed but not repeated, allowing appropriate intervals between the remaining doses.
- If the child is late for *all* immunizations, and is aged 12 months or more, the priority is to give MMR first. Polio+DTP can be given at the same time as MMR immunization, in separate injection sites *or* allow an interval of 3 weeks.

All children should be immunized, apart from the *very* few exceptions outlined below. A decision not to immunize a child is often the 'easier' choice for the professional involved but it is important to realize that it is a serious matter to withhold protection. Specialist advice (from the community physician or paediatrician) should always be sought in doubtful cases. If a child is suffering from an acute illness, consideration should be given to *postponing* the immunization. However, mild illnesses, such as upper respiratory tract infections without fever, are not contra-indications.

3 Absolute contra-indications for immunization

—Children with poor immune responses, such as those with leukaemia or other cancers, who are receiving chemotherapy, should *not* receive live virus vaccines until at least six months after the chemotherapy treatment is completed.

—Children receiving high-dose corticosteroids should not be immunized with live vaccines until three months after completion of treatment.

—If these children are in contact with measles or chicken-pox they should receive immunoglobulin as soon as possible.

—The live vaccines are: BCG, measles, polio, rubella, and MMR, but specialist opinion may recommend the administration of alternative killed vaccines. All these cases should therefore be referred for a specialist paediatric opinion.

—It is essential to ensure that siblings and close contacts of such children have received their full immunization schedule. However, these children, their siblings, and household contacts, should only receive inactivated poliomyelitis vaccine.

Pertussis

Do *not* give pertussis vaccine if there was a severe local or general reaction to a preceding dose of vaccine. The signs of a severe reaction are:

- Local reaction—redness and swelling greater than half the circumference of the limb which received the injection.
- General reaction—fever of 39.5 °C or more within 48 hours of immunization; generalized collapse; prolonged inconsolable screaming; convulsions within 72 hours of immunization.

Measles/mumps/rubella

Do *not* give MMR vaccine:

- If the child has a history of allergy to neomycin or kanamycin or a history of anaphylaxis due to any cause. This would be defined as an immediate reaction characterized by facial swelling, wheezing, stridor, and collapse. It is extremely rare. Egg allergy, as opposed to anaphylaxis, is *not* a contra-indication.
- Whilst the child is taking high-dose systemic steroids, or other immunosuppressive drugs, or is receiving X-ray therapy.
- If another live vaccine by injection has been given within three weeks.
- If the child has an acute febrile illness.

MMR vaccine should not be given within three months of an injection of immunoglobulin.

Immunoglobulin as used with measles vaccine must not be given with MMR vaccine as the immune response to rubella and mumps may be inhibited. Seek specialist paediatric advice rather than refuse vaccination.

4 Special considerations for immunization

Minor infections without a fever, particularly upper respiratory tract infections, coughs without other symptoms, and mild diarrhoea and vomiting (except with polio), are not reasons for delaying immunization.

- If the child is taking a course of antibiotics, but has no acute symptoms, do *not* delay immunization.
- If the child has an acute severe illness, especially with a fever (above 38 °C), then consider delaying immunization.

Pertussis

Refer for specialist paediatric, or community consultant opinion before a decision is made to withhold pertussis vaccine from:

- children who have had cerebral damage in the neonatal period;
- children with a history of convulsions;
- children whose parents or siblings have a history of idiopathic epilepsy.

For these children, the risk from the vaccine may be higher than normal but the effects from whooping cough disease itself could be more severe.

Neurological complications are considerably more common after whooping cough than after vaccination.

Less than 5 per cent of babies will need special consideration. A smaller percentage will have sufficient reaction to an injection to justify not completing the pertussis course.

The following are *not* contra-indications to pertussis vaccine:

- a family history of febrile convulsions;
- idiopathic epilepsy in other than first-degree relatives;
- asthma, eczema, hayfever, migraine, food allergy, other allergies in the child or child's family;
- antibiotics;
- chronic diseases, particularly heart and lung;
- failure to thrive;
- low birth weight and/or prematurity.

MMR vaccine

Children with febrile convulsions or ordinary convulsions, or whose parents or siblings have a history of idiopathic epilepsy, should be immunized against measles, mumps and rubella, but they need protection against the common, mild, febrile reaction to the injection, which can occur 7–10 days later and which may last for 2–3 days. Parents should keep a feverish child as cool as possible, and could give junior paracetamol during the 5–10 days following immunization. Parotid swelling may occur three weeks after immunization but children with such swelling are not infectious.

Immunoglobulin, as used with measles vaccine, must *not* be given with MMR vaccine, since the immune response to rubella and mumps may be inhibited. Seek specialist paediatric or community consultant advice, rather than refuse immunization.

The following are *not* contra-indications to MMR vaccine, and these children should be immunized:

- Children with severe heart or lung disease. These groups of children are especially at risk from measles disease and it is particularly important that they are immunized.
- A history of measles, mumps, or rubella, is *not* a contra-indication. In young children these diseases can be hard to diagnose. Even if the child has had the disease the vaccine is harmless.
- First-degree relatives with febrile convulsions.
- Children with personal or family history of asthma, eczema, hayfever, migraine, or food allergy.
- Child taking antibiotics, or other drugs.

If a child has been in recent contact (within 72 hours) with measles, early use of MMR vaccine may prevent the illness, but this does not apply to exposure to mumps or rubella, as the antibody response to these infections is slower.

Polio

The following are *not* contra-indications for giving polio vaccine:

- Breast-feeding—this does not interfere with the vaccine, even if a feed is given soon after the vaccine.
- Antibiotics—these do not interfere with the vaccine.
- If the baby vomits within one hour of receiving the vaccine—repeat the dose on the following day.

Offer vaccine to unimmunized relatives, by a course of three doses of oral polio vaccine at intervals of four weeks.

Special considerations

Children for whom a live vaccine is contra-indicated

Inactivated polio vaccine (IPV) should be given to children for whom a live vaccine is contra-indicated, such as those with immunosuppression from disease or therapy. IPV should also be used for siblings and household contacts, if appropriate.

HIV-positive children

These children *may* receive live polio vaccine, at the discretion of the clinician in charge, but excretion of the vaccine virus in the faeces may continue for longer than six weeks. Strict personal hygiene is advised, especially careful handwashing after changing nappies.

HIV-positive children, with or without symptoms, should receive all vaccines, *except* BCG vaccine. No harmful effects have been reported following immunization with live attenuated vaccines for measles, mumps, rubella, and polio in HIV-positive children, who may be at increased risk from these diseases.

5 Immunization procedure

History-taking

Suitability for immunization

Before the first course of immunization is given .the child must have been seen by a doctor, and found to be suitable for immunization. A prescription must then be signed by the doctor. Such a prescription can act for the whole of the primary course of immunizations. Verbal authorization may be acceptable in special situations as long as the prescription is subsequently signed.

Before each immunization the health of the child should be assessed by the health visitor or nurse, by asking the parent if the child is well, and whether she/he is happy for the immunization to go ahead.

Minor coughs or colds, or being on a course of antibiotics should not postpone immunization, but a feverish, acutely unwell child should not be immunized that day. There is no evidence that immunizing an acutely unwell child is harmful, it just makes it difficult to differentiate between a possible reaction to the vaccine, and the signs of the acute illness.

Reactions to previous immunizations

A severe reaction (see pp. 25, 26) to a previous dose of vaccine is the only absolute contra-indication for omitting subsequent doses of, for example, pertussis vaccine. The future immunization schedule for such a child should be discussed with a specialist paediatrician or community consultant.

If there has been any reaction other than a severe local or

general reaction, the child should continue with the planned immunization schedule, but where there is concern seek specialist advice.

Illness since the last immunization

If the child has developed fits, or had any serious illness or neurological symptoms since the last immunization, seek advice from the GP, specialist paediatrician, or community consultant as appropriate.

Consent

Initial written consent for inclusion on the immunization programme must always be obtained from parents or guardians.

—This written consent obtained before the giving of the immunizations is only an agreement for the inclusion of the child on the immunization programme.

—The fact that the parent then brings the child for the immunization can be seen as acceptance by the parent that the child may be immunized, if suitable.

—However, before each immunization, fitness and suitability of the child for *that* immunization must be established, and verbal consent obtained.

—Children in care may need the written consent of social services if parental consent has not been given.

Giving the immunization

Immunization by nurses

This may take place in the clinic, home, or elsewhere.

The DHSS (DHSS 1988) recommendations for immunization state:

A doctor may delegate responsibility for immunization to a nurse provided the following conditions are fulfilled:

(i)   The nurse is willing to be professionally accountable for this work.
(ii) The nurse has received training and is competent in all aspects of immunization, including the contra-indications to specific vaccines.
(iii) Adequate training has been given in the recognition and treatment of anaphylaxis.

If these conditions are fulfilled and nurses carry out the immunization in accordance with accepted District Health Authority policy, the Authority will accept responsibility for immunization by nurses.

Administration

Vaccine	Route of administration	Dose	Needle size
OPV	Oral	3 drops	Nil
IPV	Deep subcutaneous or intra-muscular	0.5 ml	23 G
D/T/P D/T	Deep subcutaneous or intra-muscular	0.5 ml	23 G
Measles Mumps Rubella	Deep subcutaneous or intra-muscular	0.5 ml	23 G
BCG	Intradermal Infants	0.1 ml 0.05 ml	25 G

OPV, oral polio vaccine; IPV, inactivated polio vaccine; D/T/P, diphtheria/tetanus/pertussis (DHSS 1988).

Procedure

—At the beginning of each session check expiry dates on the vaccines and adrenalin, and that storage conditions have been satisfactory.

—Explain to parents which vaccine is to be given and the possibility of side-effects (for advice about the management of these see p. 38).

—Check the dose name of the vaccine against the child's clinic card and draw up the vaccine immediately before administering it.

—The skin should be clean and dry before giving the immunization. If an alcohol-based swab is used, special care should be taken to ensure that the skin is dry before proceeding, as alcohol can inactivate live vaccine preparations.

—The preferred injection site for babies is the upper, outer, thigh or upper arm; and for older children, the upper, outer, arm, using an appropriate needle for a deep subcutaneous, or intramuscular injection (23 G).

—The exception to this is for BCG vaccine, which is *always* given intradermally, using a 25 G needle. The skin should be stretched between the thumb and forefinger of one hand, and the needle inserted with the other, bevel upwards, for about 2 mm, almost parallel with the skin surface. A raised, blanched bleb will appear. The injection site for BCG is over the insertion of the left deltoid muscle. For the Mantoux or Heaf test the intradermal injection site is the middle of the flexor of the forearm.

—Dispose of syringe and needle into a rigid Sharps container. **Do not resheath needles.**

—Discard opened vaccines at the end of each session. Single-dose vaccines can be ordered if necessary, for example, for a home immunization.

—When working in a clinic setting take the vaccines from the refrigerator when required. When working in any other setting, store the vaccines in a cool-bag, taking them out only when required.

Recording

It is very important that all immunizations are recorded and dated, both on the clinic cards and on health authority records.

If there are any enquiries or difficulties arising from form-filling contact:

1. _____ Tel. _____
2. _____ Tel. _____
3. _____ Tel. _____

Storing vaccines

Manufacturers' instructions for storage and reconstitution of vaccines **must** be observed.

- Vaccines must be stored in a refrigerator, but must not be kept below 0 °C.
- Reconstituted vaccines must be used within the recommended period of reconstitution, 1–4 hours according to manufacturers' instructions; all out-of-date vaccines must be discarded.
- Vaccines must be removed from the refrigerator for as short a time as possible before use: work either from the refrigerator, or the cool-bag, taking out only what is needed for each immunization.
- Vaccines must not be exposed to direct sunlight or placed near sources of heat, such as radiators.
- Any unused vaccine in multidose containers which have been opened **must** be discarded at the end of each session.

Special attention should be paid in each district to the 'cold chain' concept. This attempts to ensure that all vaccines are maintained at the correct temperature at all stages of transport and storage within the district.

Obtaining information

It is essential that parents receive correct advice. Health workers must be up to date with recent changes and recommendations, and check that their colleagues are also aware of any changes. A useful reference source is the DHSS guideline, *Immunisation against infectious disease* (1988). If a question from a parent raises uncertainties seek the correct answer *before* giving a reply.

Enquiry telephone numbers for your district are:

1. _____ Tel. _____
2. _____ Tel. _____
3. _____ Tel. _____

For enquiries about the immunization status of a child:

Tel. _____

6 Reactions to immunization

Reactions are **rare** but it is important to be aware of the possibility. Listed below are the types of reaction which may occasionally occur, and the recommended actions.

Immediate reactions

Very occasionally (approximately 1 in 300 000 administered vaccine doses), a child will collapse within seconds or minutes of being given an immunization. The exact cause of the collapse is frequently hard to ascertain, as there are difficulties in differentiating between breath-holding, vaso-vagal attacks, and anaphylactic reactions.*

The usual signs are:

- pallor
- limpness
- apnoea

If a child collapses and then rapidly recovers, this is probably a vaso-vagal or breath-holding attack. However, with anaphylaxis, in which the child may lose consciousness, or develop urticarial skin lesions, or wheezing, rapid action is required.

Action

—Ask someone to dial 999 and summon medical aid.

*American and Dutch experiences indicate that death due to anaphylaxis following immunization, if it has ever occurred, is less than 1 in 30 million doses (personal communication from Dr Renoke and Dr Salisbury to Dr Macfarlane 1988).

—Treat for shock, lie the child down, and maintain an airway.

—Administer adrenalin by intramuscular or deep subcutaneous injection, slowly, see p. 37.

—Apply cardio-pulmonary resuscitation (CPR) as necessary, and maintain until the ambulance team arrives and takes over.

—If there is no improvement in five minutes, repeat the dose of adrenalin.

—Record the reaction in the child's notes and report to the GP.

Non-specific reactions

Mild reactions

About 15 per cent of babies have a mild reaction to immunization in the first 48 hours following injection, with either some redness and soreness around the injection site or a slight fever and irritability. These mild reactions are not a contra-indication for further immunization.

Severe reactions

Very rarely, within 72 hours following immunization, a baby may have a convulsion, be extremely lethargic, or have a very red, swollen injection site around more than half the circumference of the limb.

This reaction must be reported, and if specialist medical opinion decides that it is due to pertussis immunization, rather than an intercurrent illness, then further immunizations should not contain pertussis.

Pollock *et al.* (1983) in a study of the North West Thames region found that a neurological reaction, such as prolonged febrile convulsion, may occur in approximately 1 in 100 000 children receiving a full course of D/T/P, with almost none of these suffering a long-term effect. The recent Loveday case judgment (Lancet 1988) rejected the *brain damage– pertussis vaccine* link.

Specific reactions

Mild reaction to MMR immunization

This occurs in approximately 30 per cent of children, 7–10 days after injection, and is like a very mild attack of measles, with fever, malaise, and sometimes a rash. This reaction usually lasts 24–48 hours and the vaccine virus is not transmitted to contacts. Febrile convulsions may occur, particularly if there is a simultaneous intercurrent infection, but the incidence is 8 to 10 times less than with the measles disease itself.

Mild reaction to rubella immunization

Between 3 and 10 per cent of girls may experience a mild reaction following rubella immunization, which may include fever, sore throat, rashes, and joint pains, 1–3 weeks after immunization.

7 Common problems

The child has a history of fits
Consult a specialist paediatrician before giving pertussis or measles vaccination, but no matter what type of fit it is completely safe to give polio, diphtheria, tetanus, BCG, and rubella immunizations.

A relative, other than the parents or siblings has had fits
It is safe to give all immunizations, including pertussis and measles.

The baby had neonatal problems, and was in the Special Care Baby Unit
Most of these babies should have protection from whooping cough, and for many the decision will have been taken by the time of discharge from the maternity unit and recorded in the discharge summary. If no decision has been taken, consult a specialist paediatrician about giving pertussis vaccine; it is safe to give all other immunizations.

The baby has had fits or is developing neurological problems
Refer to a specialist paediatrician for a decision about pertussis; it is safe to give all other immunizations.

The baby, or a relative, has asthma, eczema, hayfever, or other allergies
It is safe to give all immunizations, including pertussis.

The baby has a rash
Mild eczema, nappy or heat rashes, should not delay immunization.

The baby has a long-term chest or heart condition, such as cystic fibrosis, or congenital heart disease
It is safe to immunize, providing the baby is not starting or in the middle of an acute bout of illness. However, consult with the GP before delaying immunization, as THESE BABIES ARE AT PARTICULAR RISK FROM MEASLES AND WHOOPING COUGH. IT IS VERY IMPORTANT THAT THEY ARE IMMUNUIZED AS EARLY AS POSSIBLE.

The baby has been in contact with an infectious illness recently
If the baby is well, immunize.

The baby is reported to have already had the illness, such as measles and or whooping cough
Many illnesses have similar signs and symptoms and are difficult to diagnose accurately. Even if the baby has had the disease, it is safe to immunize; if the illness is misdiagnosed the baby is not left unprotected.

The baby is being given antibiotics
If the acute phase of the illness is over, it is safe to immunize. IMMUNIZATION WORKS IN BABIES AND CHILDREN TAKING ANTIBIOTICS.

The mother is breast-feeding
Immunize. BREAST-FEEDING DOES NOT INTERFERE WITH IMMUNIZATION, EVEN IF THE MOTHER IS TAKING MEDICINES.

The baby was premature: when should immunizations start?
Immunizations should start three months after the baby was born, no matter how premature.

The baby weighs under 10 lb or 4.35 kg
Immunize three months after birth, whatever the weight.

THE SMALLER THE BABY THE GREATER THE RISK IF THE
BABY CATCHES WHOOPING COUGH.

The child is aged over two years
Give any immunizations missed, including pertussis.

The child is aged over 10 years
Give any immunizations missed, except, perhaps, pertussis.
Check whether any tetanus has already been given in
casualty or by the GP.

The immunization programme has been interrupted
There is no need to start the course again. The remaining
doses should be given as if there had been no break, but if
the child is aged over 13 months start with MMR.

Giving two immunizations at once
Two live vaccines can be given simultaneously (in different
injection sites) or leave a three week gap between two live
vaccines.
     These are:

● measles,
● polio,
● rubella,
● MMR.

     BCG, also a live vaccine, *is the exception*, and should be
given alone, with an interval of three weeks before giving
another live vaccine.

The mother is pregnant
Immunizing the child will not affect the mother. It is safe to
give any immunization to the child.

The baby vomits after immunization
This is only important following polio, and only then if the

baby vomits within the first hour. If this happens repeat the dose the next day.

Children who have recently entered the country with no immunization records
Try to find out what immunizations have been given. If in doubt treat as if unimmunized and start a complete programme.

Rubella

A girl who has already had rubella
Immunize, since rubella is often misdiagnosed. It is safe to immunize a girl who has had rubella, rather than leave her possibly unprotected.

A girl who may be pregnant
Do NOT IMMUNIZE.

A woman teacher who asks to be immunized against rubella
She should consult her GP and be given a blood test to check if she is already immune. If she has no immunity, she can be immunized if she is not pregnant, and if she avoids becoming pregnant for 4 weeks following immunization.

8 Comments parents may make

There aren't many of these illnesses about these days
Measles and whooping cough are still common because our immunization uptake is poor.

Only poor children catch these illnesses
The germs can affect *any* child who is not immunized.

I'm going to keep my baby away from other children so she can't catch the germs
This won't work, because adults too can carry the germs, and sooner or later your child will meet other people.

They can treat all these illnesses these days
Babies still die from whooping cough, and there are 16–20 deaths a year amongst older children who have died of measles complications, despite having the best hospital treatment.

My child is a year old; even if he gets one of these illnesses it won't affect him much
Some of the illnesses may be serious whatever the age. Also, immunizing everyone helps to check the spread of disease and protects very young babies before they can be immunized.

I'm giving my child the homeopathic medicine against whooping cough
There is no sound evidence that this is effective. It is made from the diluted sputum of someone with whooping cough.

These immunizations don't always work
All of these immunizations provide more than 90 per cent protection if the full course is given.

Is it safer to give half a dose of immunization first?
Anything less than the full dose may not give protection. A
full dose is as safe as half a dose.

*What are the chances of my baby being brain damaged
from the whooping cough vaccine?*
In the recent Loveday case (1988) it was not proved that
whooping cough vaccine can cause permanent brain
damage. There is a much higher risk of damage from
catching the disease itself.

*Why do I need to have my child immunized if she's
already had measles, or rubella?*
Other rashes are often mistaken for measles and rubella
and it is therefore better to ensure that each child is fully
protected by immunization.

*Is it safe to take my baby swimming before he is
immunized?*
Yes, babies may be taken to public swimming pools before
receiving their first immunizations.

9 Future immunization targets

- The World Health Organization's theme for World Health Day 1987 was:

    'Immunization: a chance for every child.'

    The target is to eradicate measles by the year 2000.

- National targets for 1990 are a 90 per cent uptake for measles and pertussis.

- MMR vaccine has been introduced into the UK with the specific aim of eliminating measles, mumps, rubella and congenital rubella syndrome.

Appendix A: References and further reading

Begg, N. and White, J. (1987). *A survey of pre-school immunis-ation programmes in England and Wales.* PHLS Communicable Disease Surveillance Centre, London.

Brahams, D. (1988). Pertussis vaccine: Court finds no justification for association with permanent brain damage. *Lancet* i, 837.

DHSS (Department of Health and Social Security) (1988). *Immunis-ation against infectious disease.* DHSS, London.

DHSS (1981). In *Whooping cough: reports from the Committee on Safety of Medicines and the Joint Committee on Vaccina-tion and Immunisation.* HMSO, London.

Harvey, D. and Kovar, I. (eds) (1985). *Child health, a textbook for the DCH.* Churchill Livingstone, Edinburgh.

Hutchinson, T. *et al.* (1987). A training procedure for immunisation. *Health Trends* 19, 19–24.

Jefferson, N. *et al.* (1987). Immunisation of children at home without a doctor present. *Br. Med. J.* 294, 423–4.

Kulenkampff, M., Schwartzman, J. S. and Wilson, J. (1974). *Arch. Dis. Child.* 49, 46–9.

Lancet (1983). Failure to vaccinate. *Lancet* ii, 1343–4.

Miller, C. L. (1983). Current impact of measles in the United Kingdom. *Rev. Infect. Dis.* 5, 427–32.

Miller, C. L. *et al.* (1981). Pertussis immunisation and serious acute neurological illness in children. *Br. Med. J.* 282, 1595–7.

Nicoll, A. and Rudd, P. (1989). *British Paediatric Association Manual of Infections and Immunizations in Children.* Oxford University Press, Oxford.

Nottingham Health Authority (1985). *A practical guide to immunis-ation in children,* Nottingham Vaccination and Immunisation Committee, Nottingham.

OHE (Office of Health Economics) (1984). *Childhood vaccination: current controversies.* OHE, London.

Pollock, T. M. *et al.* (1983). A seven year study of disorders attributed to vaccination in North West Thames Region. *Lancet* **i**, 753–7.

Robertson, C. and Bennett, V. (1987). Health Visitors' views on immunisation. *Health Visitor* **60**, 221–2.

von Reyn, C. F. *et al.* (1987). Human immunodeficiency virus infection and routine childhood immunisation. *Lancet* **ii**, 669–72.

Wells, N. (1987). Immunisation—where do we go from here? In *Progress in child health* (ed. J. A. Macfarlane), pp. 60–70. Churchill Livingstone, Edinburgh.

WHO (World Health Organisation) (1985). *Targets for Health for All.* WHO, Copenhagen.

Appendix B: Child resuscitation pack

A child resuscitation pack should be available in immunization clinics and be carried by health visitors and school nurses when giving home immunizations. It should include the following:

- A box containing 2×1 ml ampoules of adrenalin 1:1000 (1 mg/ml). Instructions on the outside of the box should read:

For infants and children
Adrenalin 1:1000 (1 mg/ml).
Dose to be given slowly, over 10 to 15 seconds, intramuscularly.

Age (years)	Dose (ml)
< 1	0.05
1	0.1
2	0.2
3–4	0.3
5	0.4
6–10	0.5
11–16	0.7
Adult	1.0

(DHSS 1988.)

- 4×1 ml syringes.
- 4×23 G needles.
- Specific instruction sheet concerning the treatment of anaphylactic shock in children.
- Airway/mask suitable for children.

Appendix C: Check-list for home immunization

Each session

- Vaccine available and in date?
- Resuscitation pack available?
- Cool-bag and freezer-pack
- Syringes and 23 G needles
- Sharps box
- Sugar lumps
- Cotton wool
- Spoons
- Plasters
- Forms
- Education leaflets

Each child

- Are there any contra-indications or special considerations?
- Is the child well?
- Were there any reactions following a previous immunization?
- Are the records available, has the consent been signed, and is the parent happy for the immunization to be given?
- Define immunization to be given.
- Mention to the parents the possibility of a mild reaction.
- Tepid sponging is still advised, and the child should be kept cool, and could be offered some junior paracetamol, as well as being given lots to drink.
- Record the immunization given on all the appropriate records.

Index

adrenalin 26, 37
allergies 14, 16, 17, 28
anaphylactic reactions 14, 25–6, 37
antibiotic therapy 15, 16, 17, 29
asthma 16, 17, 28

BCG (Bacille-Calmette-Guerin)
    vaccine 8–9
    administration 21, 22
    HIV-positive children 9, 18
    immunization schedules 10, 11, 30
birth weight, low 16
brain damage
    neonatal period 15
    pertussis vaccine causing 27,
      33
breast-feeding 17, 29
breath-holding attacks 25

cancer chemotherapy 13
checklist, home immunization 38
child resuscitation pack 37
cold chain concept 24
consent, parental 20, 38
contraindications 13–14, 19–20
convulsions (fits)
    family history 16, 17, 28
    history of previous 15, 16, 20, 28
    vaccinations causing 26–7
corticosteroid therapy 13, 14
cystic fibrosis 29

diarrhoea 15
diphtheria 2–3
diphtheria/tetanus/pertussis (triple;
    D/T/P) vaccine
    administration 21
    immunization schedules 10–11
    reactions 26–7
    see also pertussis

eczema 16, 17, 28
epilepsy, family history 15, 16

failure to thrive 16
febrile illnesses, acute 14, 15, 19
febrile reactions, MMR vaccine 16, 27
fits, *see* convulsions

German measles, *see* rubella

hayfever 16, 17, 28
Heaf test 8, 9, 22
heart disease 16, 17, 29
history-taking 19–20
HIV-positive children 9, 18
home immunization, checklist 38
homeopathic medicines 32

*Immunisation against infectious
    disease* (DHSS; 1988) 24
immunization
    contraindications 13–14, 19–20
    delayed or missed 11–12, 30, 31
    history-taking 19–20
    information sources 24
    parental comments 32–3
    parental consent 20, 38
    procedure 20–3
    rationale 1–9
    reactions 19–20, 25–7
    recording 23, 38
    schedules 10–12, 30, 31
    storage of vaccines 23–4
immunoglobulin therapy
    immunosuppressed children 13
    MMR vaccination and 14, 16
immunosuppressed patients 13, 14, 18
infectious illnesses, recent contacts
    29
information sources 24

live vaccines 13, 18
lung disease 16, 17, 29

Mantoux test 8, 22

measles 5–6, 30, 34
  common problems 28–9, 30
  previous infection 17, 29, 33
  recent contact 17
measles, mumps and rubella (MMR)
    vaccine 7, 34
  administration 21
  contraindications 14
  HIV-positive children 18
  immunization schedules 10, 11, 30
  reactions 16, 27
  special considerations 16–17
migraine 16, 17
mumps 6–7, 17
  see also measles, mumps and
    rubella (MMR) vaccine

neonatal problems, history of 28
neurological illness 20, 28
  complicating pertussis
    vaccination 4, 15, 26–7
  see also brain damage; convulsions
nurses, immunization by 20–1

overseas, children from 11, 31

parents
  comments made 32–3
  consent 20, 38
  information 24
pertussis (whooping cough) 4–5,
    15–16, 34
  common problems 28, 29, 30
  contraindications 13–14
  homeopathic medicines 32
  immunization schedules 10, 11
  neurological complications 4, 15,
    26–7
  parental concerns 32–3
  severe reactions 14, 26–7
  see also diphtheria/tetanus/
    pertussis vaccine
poliomyelitis (polio) 5, 17
  administration of vaccine 21
  immunization schedules 10, 11, 30
  immunosuppressed patients 18
  inactivated vaccine (IPV; Salk) 5, 18,
    21

oral, live attenuated vaccine (OPV;
    Sabin) 5, 21
  vomiting and 15, 30–1
pregnancy 30, 31
prematurity 16, 29

rashes 28
records, immunizations 23
respiratory tract infections, upper 12,
  15
resuscitation pack, child 37
rubella (German measles) 7, 31
  congenital 7
  immunization schedules 10
  previous infection 17, 31
  reactions to vaccination 27
  see also measles, mumps and
    rubella (MMR) vaccine

schedules, immunization 10–12, 30,
  31
swimming pools, public 33

teachers, rubella immunization 31
tetanus 3
  see also diphtheria/tetanus/
    pertussis vaccine
thrive, failure to 16
triple vaccine, see diphtheria/
    tetanus/pertussis vaccine
tuberculosis 8–9

vaccines
  administration 21–3
  live 13, 18
  storage 23–4
  see also specific vaccines
vaso-vagal attacks 25
vomiting 15, 17, 30–1

weight, low body 29–30
whooping cough, see pertussis
World Health Organization 1, 34

X-ray therapy 14